Looking Back
AIDS Tales and Teachings

Looking Back
AIDS Tales and Teachings

By Jody Reiss

For all of them
and for my father, who might
have been one of them if he'd lived
in another time

Table of Contents

Introduction

It has been 40 years since the first cases of a new and deadly disease appeared. Although a variety of treatments have made AIDS a "chronic manageable illness," at least in the wealthier nations, there is still no cure. Worldwide, AIDS has killed more than 36 million people.

As the world battles the new and quickly changing pandemic of COVID-19, my thoughts return to the early days of AIDS and the people who suffered and died of the disease – their stories and lessons.

In 1983 I was getting ready to start graduate school at the University of Maryland School of Social Work after living in Maryland for several years. I had a number of friends who were gay men, and as AIDS, initially called Gay Related Immune Deficiency, began to strike closer to home, I was scared that one day one of them would get sick. I decided to begin volunteering with the Whitman-Walker Clinic in Washington, DC, and that's where I began a journey that would last for the next 18 years and would include working with several hundred people with AIDS.

For me, AIDS work was "heart and soul" work. It was about being open to forming deep and meaningful relationships, being open to falling in love, and being open to grief and withstanding it. This book combines stories and poems drawn from those relationships as well as lectures, a training, and a sermon. It looks at the lifestyles, losses, strengths, and hopes of a generation of gay men and the homophobia, fear, and blame they encountered from the world around them. It looks at the ways the professional, volunteer, and religious communities reached out to help them and, along the way, adjusted to the changing realities of the disease. In particular it looks at how the Jewish community offered culturally specific services as well as tradition and ritual to help both people with AIDS and their loved ones.

Although the names have been changed, the stories and examples in this book are all true and represent people I cared for and cared about.

2021

PART 1

TALES

The Mothers

I think about the mothers. The mothers in their small towns whose sons have left them long ago for the freedom of the city, the distance with which to hide the way they live, who they are. But the mothers, the mothers have always known; they are after all, the mothers.

Caroline stopped dead in the middle of her vacuuming as her son Jesse came through the door of the modest Tennessee farmhouse. He came to surprise her for Easter, and she was so surprised she could barely catch her breath. She just stared at him. He looked only a little paler, but otherwise no worse for the wear and tear of this disease she didn't understand and the treatment he was getting for it way up north. He was just her little boy come to surprise his mother. And then she reached for a hug.

Kerry's mother died long ago of cancer.

Wilfredo's mother came from Puerto Rico too late to find him lucid.

Brad's mother crossed over the yellow line and hit a cement truck.

Mary gave up her son for adoption, unwed mother working towards a career. But he found her 40 years later just before he was diagnosed, and she moved across the country to live with him and raise his three teenagers. As he got sicker, he talked of suicide a lot and she went out to find needles and drugs so he'd have that option. But when it came time, he didn't want to have it end that way, and Mary was hurt that he wouldn't accept her offering.

Julio's mother wasn't allowed out of El Salvador to visit him.

Tony's mother stayed with him all the time, even came to support group with him.

Dennis didn't want to tell his mother.

Melvin's mother was scared to have him in the house.

Kaye lost them both. Both her sons, boys of separate marriages, all the children she'd had. Richard, born with only one arm, growing up rebellious to become a troubled man living on the edge in New York City, hustling his body to other men, hustling drugs to anyone who'd buy. And Nick, sensitive, artistic, fighting a battle with alcohol with the help of his lover of ten years and their settled lifestyle. Never mind all the differences; both caught AIDS, and Kaye, the retired nurse, nursed them both through their final illnesses: toxoplasmosis, the same for both. And then she went home with her husband and founded the Seaside AIDS Project.

Daryl's mother came from Mississippi and cried a lot.

Kevin's mother was with him when he died in the monastery to which he'd belonged for 28 years.

Craig's mother held his hand all the several days he was on a respirator.

Teresa taught third grade in New Jersey. All that spring Jeff was bedridden, she drove the five hours down to D.C. every Friday night to spend the weekend cooking big Italian meals and coaxing him to eat, cleaning the tiny apartment, entertaining his friends. And then drove the five hours back Sunday night in time for school on Monday. In the summer she moved in for the duration. In the end he wanted to go to the beach of his childhood one last time, so her family bundled his tiny wasted body up and took him there. He got to see the boardwalk once more before he died in his mother's arms early in August.

1986

He Might Have Been Queen

He was tall, very tall. And he was wearing cowboy boots, which made him taller. But he was thin already, thin and delicate, and he walked as if every bone ached. He had a pretty face, soft green eyes, and clear, soft skin. His hair was brown and he wore it short and conservative, but you could see in the back how he was letting it grow into a tail, which was the style at the time. His moustache was thin and it did not look as if he could grow a beard. In his left ear were two rather large diamond studs.

He had rung the bell and I'd come down the steps to meet him and to take him through the clinic to the basement, which hopefully would offer us a private place to talk. We settled into a waiting area at the front of the building, Brad easing himself gingerly into his seat. We were at the end of a hallway with little rooms on either side. Some were very small and were used for interviewing. Their walls were covered with posters proclaiming the ten warning signs of gonorrhea and what you should know about the Hepatitis B vaccine. On the other side of the hall were three examining rooms with examining tables and containers of Vaseline and tubes of KY jelly lying about. I'd opted for the less private open space of the waiting room. VD Clinic was only open in the evening.

That's how I met Brad, that's how we started. We started with the disease, with when he'd been diagnosed, with the Pneumocystis and the shots of pentamidine that had made his butt all lumpy. We talked about the nurse coming in three times a week to give him more shots, of streptomycin for the suspected myobacterium avium-intracellulare. There were lots of complicated medical terms like that that Brad seemed to take pleasure in pronouncing properly, as if he'd known them all his life.

And then the gears switched, and Brad asked, "Do you think it's okay to want to die?" Caught off guard, I reacted out of habit, "Do *you* think it's okay?" Without a moment's hesitation, Brad shot back, "Don't give me that shit, that's what my psychiatrist tells me."

* * * * * * * * *

"Hives, temperature 104.4, reaction, Resterol, hives, cold ice pack." These were the words I wrote in my notebook as I sat at the clinic talking on the phone. Brad was too sick to come see me that day, too sick to have remembered our counseling appointment. When I called him at noon I woke him up. He was feeling sorry for himself. Lonely. "Are you good at jigsaw puzzles? Maybe you could come over and do one with me sometime."

Brad wanted to go home. Home to Saginaw, Michigan, might be the last time. He had it all planned. "I've got an ulterior motive for going home," he began. "I want to wreck someone's nerves. She's a drag queen, actually a transsexual who's having some real problems with the change. I made the mistake of telling her I have AIDS and she went and told everyone. There's only one bar in Saginaw. You gotta drive a hundred miles to find another gay bar where everyone doesn't know you." He was talking slow, with the anger building slowly in his voice. "She's doing a show February 14 and I'm planning a little surprise. I'm going to take my fur and my sequins and my dark makeup, drop some coins on stage and tell her what she can do with them."

* * * * * * * * *

I'm scanning the horizon
for someone recognizing
that I might have been queen

Those lines are from a song Tina Turner sang, and when I hear them on the radio, I think of Brad up on a little stage mouthing along.

Brad did go to Saginaw that February and came back spent and run-down from the traveling and the strange bed and the streptomycin shots from a strange doctor. He walked slowly, buckling a little now and then at the knees, as he entered the room where we held support group. He had arrived early and he sat on a hard green folding chair under a bank of fluorescent lights, waiting for the others. As they arrived one by one, men of different ages and different stages of health, he directed them to look through the stack of photographs he'd brought. Each man in turn was drawn into the mood, and the room became animated with questions and laughter and exclamations of "Is that really you?"

In one of the photos Brad was on stage holding a cordless microphone to his mouth with long thin fingers that ended in long thin fingernails painted bright red. His moustache was gone and his smooth skin was a shade or two darker than its natural color. He wore a black wig with waves of thick hair cascading below his shoulders, hair that was coarse and full the way Black women's hair is after it's been straightened. He wore a blue shirt tied at the waist and a very tight, very short, black leather mini-skirt. He wore black nylons on his tremendously long legs and six-inch red platform pumps. Although he bore no obvious resemblance to her, except perhaps for the length of his legs, this had been Brad's outfit for his Tina Turner numbers.

After the excitement died down about the photographs Brad had brought, he sat quietly holding them in his lap. He pulled the cap he wore so often over his eyes as if to let us know that the show was over, he had nothing more to say. Around his neck was a gold chain with a gold pendant spelling out a single word: *STAR*.

* * * * * * * * *

Money was not one of Brad's concerns. At 29 he had put in ten years as a telephone operator and was enjoying liberal disability benefits. He had started working for the phone company in Saginaw, back when he had been married. His ex-wife had since become a race-car driver and he was fairly sure she was a lesbian.

Brad had been living with his lover, a man 15 years his senior and one of the first Black men to have been an umpire for National League Baseball. The two men fought often, sometimes coming to blows, and when I met Brad, they were in the midst of one of their periodic separations. "Now when he comes to visit," said Brad, "he sleeps on the davenport. The first time, well okay, so he fell asleep watching TV. But after six times I get the picture." His voice had gotten soft and he stared at his hands, "I miss the sex, but mostly I miss the touch."

* * * * * * * * *

Brad's mother was killed in a car accident. "It was on the news." He'd moved to Washington in November, didn't go home for Christmas. When he went home the end of January, he got into town late so he stayed over with some friends. The next morning his mother went to pick up her sister Cindy and Cindy's twins, crossed over the yellow line and hit a cement truck. "You should have seen her casket," said Brad, "red velvet for days. Mom loved red. I put a red carnation on her grave every time I go. But sometimes when I'm trying to remember a recipe, I'll call her up and be shocked again that she's not there."

* * * * * * * * *

At the end of May Brad was in the hospital, severely dehydrated from intestinal parasites destroying his body's ability to absorb fluid. I arrived one morning in a rush from a tight schedule and upcoming vacation and made my way to Brad's room on the third floor. On the door was a blue and red sign announcing, "Blood and Body Fluid Precautions."

Inside, Brad was bundled up under several blankets, shivering from the cold of a phantom fever. Only his thin, tired face was visible, and I thought his watery big green eyes looked very scared and very vulnerable. Brad was tired. This visit, he did not ask me to close the door so he could smoke a cigarette without the nurses knowing. I sat in a chair on one side of the bed and asked him what was left undone. "I want to see my cats again. You could probably sneak Dog in, but Brutus would put up such a fuss that everyone would know."

We talked of his desire to go home and of his fear and of how complicated it would be now that the doctor had started hyperalimentation – the form of complete nutrition pumped through a tube in his chest to the vein just outside the heart. And then gently I said, "I'm going to have to leave in a minute." And gently Brad pleaded, "So soon?" and began to cry. I stood then and went to the bed, and as I held his head I began to cry, too. With great effort he wrestled his long thin arms free from the blankets and the chest tube and the IV and wrapped them around me to hold me close as we both cried. Cried in a silence that soon became too painful, and so I said, "I'm really going to miss you, Brad." "Not so fast," he replied as he mustered his strength to break the spell and push me away, "I'm not going anywhere."

* * * * * * * * * *

Brad did go somewhere, he went home. And one Sunday night I received a call from Tony, the nurse who was living in.

"Could you bring a wheelchair when you come tomorrow, Brad wants to go to group."

There weren't very many of us that night. Besides me and the man I led group with, there were only Stan and Jim and Wilfredo, three old-timers like Brad who had been diagnosed about the same time and who were declining at a similar rate.

I heard the door and I turned to see Tony and another man pushing Brad towards us. After getting him settled, they quickly retreated. Brad was pale and so terribly winded, it took him nearly half the session to catch his breath, gather his strength enough to speak. He wore an army fatigue shirt, which he slowly unbuttoned so that it fell open, revealing the hyperalimentation leads where they entered his chest. He sat all hunched over, occasionally taking a sip from the straw of the 7UP sitting in his lap.

"I'm stopping the hyperal on Friday," Brad said finally. "My insurance will only pay for three weeks at home. It's the only thing keeping me alive and it's not enough." The room was silent as he shifted his weight in his chair. "I'll die anyway with it, but without it the doctor says I'll only have a few days. So, I wanted to come and tell you guys how much you've meant to me."

We were silent awhile. And then Jim spoke: "Well, you sure picked a dignified way to do it." "I thought I owed it to you," said Brad, "to at least say it in person." At this Jim was up and across the room, bending down and gently giving Brad a hug, "I love you, kid." After a minute or two, Stan asked, "Are you tired, you want to go home now?" and went off to find Tony.

* * * * * * * * * *

Brad used to bring me flowers every week he was able to come in to the office, nothing too fancy but every bouquet different and every bouquet resilient enough to last the week through on my desk at home until they were replaced the next week.

One day in early April Brad had arrived looking particularly pale and weak. But his bouquet was vibrant with red roses, white carnations, and bright purple straw flowers. As I admired the flowers he said, "If you hang the purple ones upside down and let them dry, they'll last forever." I kept that sprig of purple flowers for nearly a year after Brad died, two or three months after he brought them to me, the last day he was strong enough to come to the clinic to meet me.

Brad died at 30 in 1985

For Tom

Doesn't matter how tough you are

How much leather you've worn

How many men you've had in your

    rough and angry way

Doesn't matter how nasty you can be

In your frustration and your pain

Refusing all your favorite food

Any food

Doesn't matter that you won't take the morphine

Rather to toss and turn and know

    you are alive

Doesn't matter

When you die you're like a baby again

And we hold you softly in our arms

    Tom died at 38 in 1985

Such A Lovely Time

"Tennessee?" comes the incredulous voice of my father over the phone from San Francisco, "but nobody goes to Tennessee. I don't even know where Tennessee is." Being my father's daughter, I share in a certain amount of incredulity myself for my upcoming excursion. "Well, I know," I respond, "but I'm going. It's not so far from Washington and Jesse wants to surprise his mother for Easter."

I had met Jesse six months earlier at a party for the Clinic in D.C. I was there because the first person with AIDS I'd volunteered with had died the day before and I wanted to be around people who had known him. The party was in the afternoon on the third floor of a Dupont Circle bar with a tastefully catered buffet. The guests were a mix of Clinic staff, volunteers like me, and the more prominent patients – Jeff, insisting that I be able to describe my mood as more than just "okay" considering how close I had been to the deceased, and Karen, arriving grandly attired in a full-length fox-fur coat with little fox heads and tails attached, commenting to me that she'd need to buy a new black hat for this latest funeral coming up.

After a time, I spotted Greg in the crowd and made my way to him, balancing a plate of raw vegetables and little spinach pies. He was the vice president of the Clinic and we were on a county committee together, but I knew him best through a mutual friend who had introduced us at a Halloween party where Greg had been in full drag. Greg was standing with a wiry young man with sharp Anglican features – this was Jesse – who held his body tight, as if ready to strike while he observed the room. He had short brown hair and a trim brown mustache and he was dressed in the uniform of the day – flannel shirt and tight jeans – only his hair was a little too long and his jeans just a bit too short to make him a perfect clone. What he lacked in gay chic fashion sense, he more than made up for with the sparkle in his soft brown eyes. I was charmed at once, even before Greg said, "There's someone I'd like you to meet."

The three of us chatted for a few minutes about the food and the Clinic and some man across the room who'd caught Jesse's eye and then Greg put his arm around my shoulder and said, "I think you should be Jesse's case manager." I was stunned. Case managers were volunteers for people who died horrible deaths and who looked ugly and miserable while doing so, as I'd so recently witnessed. This charming picture of health bore no resemblance to . . . "Oh my God, not him too," I thought, but recovered my composure without skipping a beat. "Well, certainly, if that's what he wants." But it wasn't.

Jesse and I excused ourselves to talk awhile about his situation. He was in town to be part of an NIH study using alpha-interferon and so far, he was in total remission from Kaposi's sarcoma and doing fine. He was working for the Clinic now as a peer counselor and "gal Friday." I was willing to accept him at his word when he said, "I don't need a case manager," but then he added mischievously, "Besides, I don't think anyone could keep up with me."

* * * * * * * * *

I look across at him now, across the long red plush front seat of his big American Buick and smile as I remember that first meeting. We are making our way through the empty early Saturday morning streets of Washington, D.C. headed for 95 South. Just outside the city I put a tape on and Jesse lights up a joint. "I hope you don't mind," he says, "it's going to be a long nine hours and this is the way I like to do it." I tell him, "fine by me" but I won't be joining him; I stopped doing grass years ago when I found it didn't always agree with me. We continue on, mostly in silence except for me singing along to the tapes I'd mixed.

After a few hours Jesse lights up again and this time my resistance, weak from the start, is shot all to hell and I toke along. Our conversation picks up after that and so does the vehemence with which I belt out the tunes, from Baez to the Pointer Sisters, whose "Jump" is one of Jesse's current favorites.

Just outside Roanoke Jesse pulls over, spreads his grandmother's patchwork quilt in a field, puts some Mozart on the boom box, and serves up a gourmet meal on real plates – marinated mushrooms and chicken breasts stuffed with artichokes, asparagus, and cashews kept warm since early morning, wrapped in gingham dish towels. And big beautiful strawberries for dessert.

* * * * * * * * * *

Our first meal together had not been so elaborate. Six weeks after I'd met Jesse, I found myself sitting in a booth with him at a cheap Chinese restaurant on "P" Street. At dinner I learned how he'd been what was then called pre-AIDS for a year and a half, waiting tables at the Peachtree Plaza and doing volunteer work for AID Atlanta. When they found KS lesions on his gums, the diagnosis came mostly as a relief. Jesse seemed proud and defiant about his lifestyle, which had included a former habit of shooting methedrine. "You know that cover of Time that shows the man with a thousand sex partners. Well, that's me, really it ought to be anyway. I'm him." Even as I felt a bit put off by the lifestyle, I was drawn in by Jesse's pride and by how hard he was going to fight to maintain that pride, and I was energized by his sparkle.

From the restaurant we proceeded to the Lost and Found, across town in a district that pulsed with the hard work of the warehouse by day and the gay disco by night. The place was packed but we quickly found a spot on the dance floor. Jesse had a nice style to his step, but mostly he held his upper body stiff, with his fists out in front of him lightly clenched, as if ready to duke it out with anyone who crossed his path. I danced feverishly, changing my step often to try to follow his moves. Mostly his attention was taken up by his survey of the crowd, but occasionally our eyes met, and those few moments of connection were enough for me to feel a sense of sadness and to think, "Here's when my heart starts to break." As we stepped off the dance floor, Jesse said soberly, "You've got the job. Your first assignment as my case manager is to help this Southern boy come up with a winter wardrobe."

* * * * * * * * *

Jesse slows the Buick as we enter the only town in the South known to have fought on both sides of the Civil War and displaying statues to that effect in its town square. His parents live on a farm 20 miles outside of town. As we round the final bend, he starts honking the horn wildly - "tradition," he tells me. Even so, his parents aren't prepared; his mother stops dead in the middle of her vacuuming as we walk through the door. No tears, but after a long stare, an even longer hug.

I am exhausted. The drive, the feast, but mostly the marijuana, have left me grateful for the bedroom I am now shown to. The room is long and narrow and sits on the side of the house away from the road. It was Jesse's room growing up and the four-poster bed is where he was found having sex with another boy at 17. I feel both honored and uncomfortable to be here at the site of such an intimate and momentous incident in his life. I lie down but find sleep slow in coming, as I review the past events that have brought me to this room.

* * * * * * * * * *

I had become Jesse's case manager in December, a role characterized by its vagueness – "You'll do anything from cleaning his toilet to becoming his best friend," volunteers were told in training. Our first days of getting to know each other were spent shopping – turtlenecks and sweaters and black boots so cute I bought a matching pair. When we were tired, we'd stop for exotic coffees at a little shop in White Flint Mall where the copper-covered tables made Jesse's face glow with warmth.

In January Jesse and I started working side by side at the Clinic where I was doing a social work internship. On Monday nights, before the support group he attended and the other one that I led, we'd sample the various cuisines up and down 18th Street in the Adams Morgan neighborhood. He decided that eating with his fingers at the Ethiopian place, the Red Sea, was barbaric, and I found he had a stronger stomach than I for the cheap food at the Mexican dive. Meanwhile, his remission held and a gastrointestinal series in February found him completely cancer-free.

Jesse was having fun, meeting new people everywhere who seemed always to treat him well, playing up his role as Clinic mascot. During those months he phoned me every day, just checking in, just telling me of a new escapade or a new boyfriend. In the bars he was always being asked home and before accepting he'd ceremoniously disclose his ailment and lay down the rules. He never once was turned down. I found more and more that I'd wait for his calls, though when they came, they were brief and insubstantial. He left messages on my machine like, "Ziggy Stardust here. Talk to you later." Most times I felt like Mom, and, like Mom, was glad to see him happy.

* * * * * * * * * *

Under an unfamiliar patchwork quilt, I doze off and wake in a fog. From outside the bedroom door Jesse's mother is calling softly, "You better start getting' ready, dear." "Okay, thanks," I yell. It's time for the church barbecue down at Glenwood High School, and I'm hoping a quick shower will clear my head first. It doesn't, but it doesn't seem to matter. There is little conversation during the slow car ride, so I let my mind wander up and down the landscape, and when we get to the school, no one pays any particular attention to me. The event is held in the cafeteria, which doubles as a gymnasium. Women with hair nets and clear plastic gloves dish out portions of pork or beef barbecue served on a bun with coleslaw and potato chips. We sit at long picnic-style tables and every few minutes someone – cousin, neighbor, friend – approaches Jesse with a surprised welcome and a clap on the back.

Soon dinner is over and we are back at the house, shivering on the back porch as we watch Jesse's niece and nephew show off what they've been learning in dance class. After a time, Jesse's mother puts on her clogging shoes and joins them. Later in the house she and Jesse have an animated conversation about square dance steps. She doesn't realize that the "girls" he dances with are mostly men who are arbitrarily given pink bandanas to wear around their necks when they enter the Western bar he frequents.

Easter morning. I awake after the parents have left for church, but before Jesse is up. I wander through the quiet house, curious for its secrets. In the living room I encounter an enormous RCA television console that was presented to Jesse's father on the occasion of his retirement after 35 years with the company. In the den is a framed picture of Jesse's older brother Wayne with the inscription, "In appreciation for the educational opportunities you have given me." Sitting on the music stand of the Hammond organ are copies of The Methodist Hymnal and The Chancel Choir. Except for the volume of Bloom County cartoons Jesse has brought along, these are the only two books I find in the house.

By now I can hear Jesse stirring and soon he emerges, groggy from the NIH-supplied sleeping pills he's gotten in the habit of taking. He takes me out in the family pickup truck to see his land, acres and acres of rolling hills the color of moss, their definition softened by a light mist. We park, light a joint, and start walking back towards a little glen where Jesse says he's always wanted to build a log cabin.

By the time we're back to the house, it has started to rain softly, but Jesse isn't finished yet. "You want country?" he asks with an exaggerated twang, "I'll give you country." And with that he opens up the barn doors, pulls out the tractor, perches me on top, and takes pictures for my family in California.

Easter dinner is at noon and I meet all the cousins and their kids, the aunts and the uncles that I hadn't already met at the barbecue. Jesse keeps disappearing with different cousins for heart to hearts out by the barn. A couple of them have survived bouts with cancer, and since that's what they think he has, they figure he can survive it too. No one treats us like a couple. Mostly no one questions my presence, but one cousin asks Jesse what I do for a living and another asks if I have cancer too.

* * * * * * * * * *

The beginning of March, Jesse had become the first resident of the new housing facility run by the Clinic. When he moved in, I gave him a black teapot and little pink cups, because he had said how much he'd missed serving tea all those months he'd lived in a hotel room paid for by NIH. That night I took him to a performance of Bach's Mass in B Minor at the Kennedy Center because he had professed love for, though ignorance of, classical music. He wore the grey pants my parents had sent during our winter shopping spree, a white shirt and a red bow tie, and he turned not a few heads.

* * * * * * * * * *

We get back to D.C. around midnight and Jesse pulls up to my house to drop me off. It's all I can do to stumble out of the car and into the house, where I fall into bed for the next 24 hours. Jesse, on the other hand, is glad to have made such good time on the road and to still have a couple hours of good dancing time left, so off he goes, kiss on the check, "such a lovely time."

Jesse died at 29 in 1986

Reggie

It's hard to remember now why he was always yelling at me. Reggie had a unique brand of denial that translated into having no insight whatsoever. Everything bad that happened to him, which was almost everything altogether, was someone else's fault, and he was real good at articulating just what that fault was all about. Sometimes I'd get caught in the crossfire and I'd hold the phone at arm's length while he'd yell and yell and slowly wind himself down enough to just talk. I guess he yelled at me because there really was no one else.

Reggie was so out of place in his world, I often wondered how he'd survived. A screaming queen in a violent Black neighborhood where every block sported a crack house. He was beating the odds – a Black man still alive at 28 in a neighborhood where most didn't hit 25, a Black man alive with AIDS for two years at a time when Black men with AIDS in Maryland weren't expected to live more than nine months.

It wasn't as if his family knew those statistics, but somehow they'd given up on him anyway after about a year, like it was time. I remember driving him to the emergency room of the county hospital once because he couldn't breathe, only time he ever let me touch him, holding his hand in the crowded hallway while he lay feverish on a gurney.

His mom and aunt came that time, sauntered in after Reggie and I had been there awhile, no sign of alarm on their faces, weary after doing battle so long with Reggie's illness and their own illnesses and addictions. They sat in the waiting room watching TV and left me to sit with Reggie. Somehow when I left, I knew they'd just stay there, watching TV and drinking coffee, while Reggie stayed alone, shivering on that gurney.

* * * * * * * * * *

Sometimes when Reggie got angry, he was right: in fact, he had an uncanny way of knowing just how to get to me and break me down so I'd end up feeling incompetent and unprofessional. I had bought a new car, a sporty Honda CRX I was thrilled with, five-year loan payment notwithstanding. A co-worker had given me a bumper sticker for it – "Fight AIDS, Not People with AIDS" – and I'd proudly affixed it to my rear bumper.

Then one day I went to pick up Reggie to take him to a court hearing about paternity payments for a child he'd fathered in a drunken haze and futile effort to prove his heterosexuality. I could have let him take the long bus ride that would leave him off a half a mile short, but I had the time and it figured into a concept of holistic client services. I parked out in front of the run-down two-story corner house with peeling yellow paint and a few boarded-up windows. It was cleaner than it had been, since Reggie had complained to the landlord that one of the roommates was smoking crack all the time and had gotten kicked out.

I knocked. When Reggie came out, he took one look at the new car and the new message and pushed me quickly inside the car – "Go, get going" he started to yell. "Don't you ever park in front of my house again. You park down the street. Bad enough, Black man and a white woman, bad enough without you go telling everybody my business."

* * * * * * * * * *

It's hard to remember now all the ways Reggie could get to me. Everything was always urgent with him; I remember that. One day he called me in a panic because Medical Assistance was about to cut him off; I must look into it immediately, it was life and death. So, I'd jumped in, made a half-dozen calls to incompetent, petty bureaucrats lording their petty power over me until I had an answer. Then I'd called Reggie back and he'd been totally disinterested, as if it had never mattered in the first place.

* * * * * * * * * *

One day in December I went to see Reggie in a double room in the county hospital. He always complained so much about any roommate that the staff had learned to put him alone if at all possible. Before I'd barely said hello, he started. "Could you pour me some more water? No, no, just half a cup. Could you pull that curtain closed? No, no, further. No, a little less." He had me running and we didn't talk, certainly not the about the reason I was there, which was to say goodbye since I was moving back to the West Coast. "Roll the blanket down. No, no, roll it, don't fold it." Awkwardly I tried to tell him that I'd miss him, that I was sorry I was leaving, while he nodded a bit and stared out the window. But as I bent down for a brief hug, he reached up and kissed me on each cheek. And when I was almost out the door, he called after me, "Throw a rose off the Golden Gate Bridge and think of me."

I last saw Reggie in 1989

In the Stillness of a Sex Club

Robert lay in the county nursing home, confined to his bed, his eyes opening and closing oblivious to the sunlight streaming in the window, body indifferent to the ward cats who would occasionally jump on the bed, hair grown into soft blond curls, and mouth silent nearly all the time now. It was late afternoon and the nurse said he hadn't spoken all day.

He was just a boy really when I met him, a cocky British boy with a Cockney accent, a shaved head, John Lennon glasses, a black leather jacket with a silver cock ring in the right epaulet, bad skin, and teeth formed into a rather prominent overbite. I confess that at first, I wasn't sure what to do with him.

I decided I would put him in my support group, a group of seven other men with AIDS who had been meeting for several months. He was the youngest by several years, with the oldest men old enough to be his father and then some. As became clear rather quickly, he was also the only one of them who had much of a sex life, at least the kind of wild life that got him entrapped by a police officer in the bushes at Land's End. In group he was wild and sullen and petulant, coming late almost every week so he'd miss everyone else's check-in but still have time for his own rambling tales of adventure. The others tolerated him or ignored him, a few got very close to him – I thought of them collectively as the "bad boys" – but eventually, after a little over a year, his lack of responsibility and commitment to the group led them to oust him. But before that he always had a story to tell. He seemed to have an insatiable need to entertain and shock that was eclipsed by a greater need to be accepted. It was hard sometimes to see him work at such cross-purposes with his own desires.

Robert had grown up in an observant Jewish home in London. His father had been a businessman who had parlayed a small import/export business in England into a larger one in Australia and eventually New Zealand before returning home to start his family. Robert's mother had died when he was nine, but soon enough he'd acquired a wicked stepmother and a pair of twin brothers whom he doted on. He was sent to private schools while his older sister bitterly attended public schools. When he was 18 his father died, and it was at this point that Robert rebelled against what had been a confining assumption that he would grow up to take his father's place heading the business. He plunged headlong into gay life in the East End, taking on the clothing, the accent, and the swagger of his new working-class companions.

He came to this country on a tourist visa, came to San Francisco for the best AIDS care in the world. He used an alias when he signed up for services and made sure to leave and return to the country every six months to keep his visa current. He knew the games to play in a country inhospitable to people with HIV. He'd been an HIV counselor himself in London and knew quite a lot about how to get what he wanted. Once he was admitted to the emergency room with a fever of 103 and an infection in the catheter used to receive twice daily infusions. He'd had the catheter, a portacath, installed in London, and when they tried to replace it with a cheaper Hickman line he threw such a fit that they relented.

Robert settled into a group house in the Haight with six roommates and went about sampling all the varied and diverse aspects of gay culture he could fit into his schedule. But as his exploration progressed, so too did his illness, and soon he was losing vision so fast that even his closest friend refused to ride on the back of his motorcycle any longer. It was at this point that Robert decided to take a trip – New Zealand, where he planned to go bungee jumping off a cliff, Australia for Mardi Gras, and

England. I think the day we said good-bye neither of us were sure he'd be back.

But, sure enough, two months into his trip, I received a postcard of a kangaroo on a surfboard that read: "So much for Mardi Gras! I spent three weeks in hospital in Sydney with a CMV flare-up, which involved losing a chunk of sight. Nevertheless, I'm in surprisingly good spirits, having met some lovely and sexy people and enjoying Sydney."

And sure enough, a few weeks later he was back. Not long after he returned, he lost the final bit of his sight. In those days blindness usually came at the end of one's disease. Few people made much attempt to adjust, and gave in without a passing thought to a cane or Braille or indicators for the knobs on the stove so one could tell how high the flame was turned up. Robert didn't let go so easily. He made an incredible adjustment to using the cane. He would come to see me and would refuse my help down the long hallway when he was leaving. I'd anxiously peer out of my office and watch as he'd hit one wall, overcompensate and hit another, get tangled up with the Xerox machine, and finally be escorted to the stairs by a helpful colleague. How he managed out in the world I never knew.

In fact, Robert's blindness did usher in the end of his life. In rapid succession he came down with a series of infections that took away his strength. As I anticipated, our meeting at the nursing home was our last and he died the following week.

His grieving friends and roommates went into high gear to create the kind of memorial that would best honor him. In keeping with how he lived his life, the service was held in the upstairs room of a sex club in the early evening before opening hours.

The walls were covered with black and white photos of Robert posing bald and naked in a graveyard, a video showed him camping it up in drag, and a tape played of him chanting prayers at his bar mitzvah. Candles were lit, words were said, the Kaddish was recited. And then those assembled began to tell stories, dozens and dozens of stories, each more poignant and hilarious than the one before and each capturing some aspect of Robert perfectly.

I had not expected to say anything, did not think I had a story to tell that would leave people nodding their heads thinking, "That's just like him." And then I remembered our good-bye. For a few moments I was back in that sunny hospital room staring at his silent mouth and unseeing eyes. I pushed a cat off the chair by his bed, sat down and took his hand. It's not a comfortable thing saying good-bye as a monologue, and soon I was on my feet again. This time I stroked his curly blond hair and said, "Who would have thought, who would ever have thought that such a tough guy as you would end up being so pretty."

He turned his face toward me then and said in a full voice, "Oh, I'm very eclectic," and then his head fell back on the pillow and he was silent once again.

Robert died at 26 in 1992

The Bridge

I am parked overlooking the ocean

as it gathers to become the bay.

It's a dreary afternoon,

rain turning to drizzle turning to calm again.

And as I look across at the cars crossing the bridge,

I too feel my calm shatter and churn

and then subside again to calm.

What were his thoughts as he drove?

What was he wearing?

Old tattered clothes, expendable,

or the new ones he'd just bought that spring?

Did he have on sexy underwear?

Did he carry some small memento

of Israel, the university and the army and the Israeli lover?

of the DC internship, the organizing of tens of

      thousands to come and march?

of San Francisco, the tiny urban park he grew with stolen water

      until the city gave in and saw that it blossomed?

And when he parked, was his mood gloomy or defiant?

Did he walk quickly looking over his shoulder,

or stroll, taking in each sensation?

Was he calm, was he angry, did he cry?

Was he proud, a hero's pride?

And how long did he stand looking out at the city?

Did he smile, say a prayer, ask forgiveness?

For someone with AIDS who died by suicide at 33 in 1993

Epitaph

They buried Josh today in a plain pine box in a plot right up against the wall on the other side of a noisy suburban thoroughfare. An indigent burial, a witnessed burial; only I was the only witness.

I'd arrived at the Jewish cemetery about 10 after 2; they were there waiting for me even though I was 20 minutes early. There had been a funeral at 1, and I suppose it had gone like clockwork and now they were anxious to get on with things. I parked a short distance away and walked along a small road to where they were waiting.

Standing beside the hearse was a large man in an oversized black felt fedora and a black double-breasted suit. He held out a beefy hand to shake mine and said in a solemn voice, "Hello; Jack Shanahan. Would you like us to go ahead and place the coffin in the grave?" I nodded.

Jack and another man from the Jewish funeral home, about half Jack's size and clearly straining from the task, and the two Latino cemetery workers took the coffin from the hearse and walked the short distance to the grave. There they laid it on some boards and thick fabric straps, which they used to lower it as they withdrew the boards.

Perhaps they had expected more people. They had unfolded a contraption into three green canvas chairs with metal arms dividing them. I chose to stand. Jack reached over to one of the shovels stuck in the pile of dirt from the grave and handed it to me. Then all four of them retreated a short distance.

I'd expected to be sad, I'd been sad for days, but all I could think of was that I should act quickly because it was Friday afternoon and I figured these guys wanted to go home. I took the shovel and performed an age-old ritual: I dug into the soft moist earth and toppled a shovelful of dirt onto the casket below. I'd seen this ritual dozens of times when a mother, most often on the frail side trying hard to hold up, had been handed a shovel to throw dirt on a son's coffin. It always made me cry. But after she was done, there would be the shovelfuls of tens of dozens of friends and family and business associates and fellow congregants and acquaintances, so that by the time the funeral party had left, the cemetery workers had an easy time filling in the rest. The whole community shared the task of burying its dead, and here I was alone with this enormous responsibility.

My shovelful of dirt was not very large, but what I couldn't manage in muscle power for shoveling, I knew I could manage with my voice. First I recited the *Kaddish*, the prayer for the dead so ancient it is not in Hebrew, but in ancient Aramaic, and then I sang, or rather chanted, *El Maleh Rachamim*, a beautiful prayer asking God to take this soul up in the bonds of life and shelter him beneath God's wings. But I was self-conscious. Could they all hear me or was my prayer muffled in the traffic from El Camino Real? Did they find the chant interminable? Did they care?

I blew Josh a kiss and turned to walk away. Jack joined me and said in a congenial way, "It's hard, but someone has to do it." But then to make sure he hadn't made a mistake, he asked if I was a relative. After I explained the circumstances, that no, I was his social worker, he said, "Yeah, the mortuary makes sure they get a proper burial." But who were the "they?" The indigent versus the "digent?" The Jews versus the non-Jews? I decided that for Jack the difference between us and them was that we, the undead, don't need burial just yet.

When I had called the Indian woman at the hotel where Josh lived, she said, "He died? Why did he die?" My mind went into overdrive – why? Because there isn't any good alcoholism treatment, because he fell through every crack the system had, because no one knew how to help him, because no one loved him. And then I realized she didn't mean why, but how, and I told her about the fall and hitting his head and the surgery. What I didn't tell her was about the call from General Hospital – Josh must have kept my card in his wallet – and how they asked me if they could pull the plug since there was no hope and no next of kin. How I agonized over it for just a brief time and never even told my supervisor before telling them to go ahead. It wouldn't have made much difference, days versus hours, already brain dead.

Josh's file at the agency was thick, thick and sloppy with entries jotted down quickly by dozens of different hands, mostly illegible. He was a frequent walk-in client who was usually seen by the "social worker of the day," but I had requested that I be called first if he showed up, trying to offer a bit of consistency. I knew he'd been a client for years, 16 to be exact, but it wasn't until after he died and the mortuary and the medical examiner's office were full of questions that I paid attention to the label on his file: "2 of 2." That meant there was a 1 of 2 somewhere, and I became obsessed for a few days with finding it. The woman in accounting called closed storage for me, but after a thorough search, they came up cold, so I was told it must have been destroyed. This was proper procedure for an out-of-date file, someone we hadn't seen for seven or eight years, but Josh had never been out of date. I knew 2 of 2 got started because 1 of 2 got too full. What was in there? I knew Josh had told previous workers he had left home at 17 to join the Marines, but there was no evidence he had done so. If I knew that I'd have some key to when his problems started. Was he developmentally delayed, schizophrenic, or suffering from alcohol psychosis? All had been diagnosed at different times during the last 16 years, but the key to which one was true lay, I was sure, in 1 of 2. Somehow it seemed terribly important to me then, even as he lay in the morgue, to be able to shed light on his life and how it had gone so wrong.

Or was it so wrong? He had his strengths. He had a capacity to maintain a stable living situation, even if that was a single room in a Tenderloin hotel. He had the freedom not to bathe or cut or comb his hair, to buy vodka at the Safeway instead of food, to isolate himself. I came across an entry in his file as part of an assessment for Social Security disability describing Josh's pastimes. It read like an epitaph: "Josh reads science fiction, draws pictures of airplanes and buses, wanders the streets, and occasionally goes to an action movie."

Josh died at 37 in 1996, not from AIDS

David

In most cases I wasn't there for the dismantling of memories, the stuff of dead people, treasured objects stripped of their meaning now that their owner has passed on, the itemization and separation of the junk from those things which hold value for family or others.

But I was there for David. He was just 25. He had lived in a small room in a small flat on Cortland Avenue and he died so quickly his father missed his final days. The father came afterward, handsome, blond, not yet 50, beaten down but trying to remain stoic for his young son, David's 5-year-old half brother he'd brought with him.

We stood in David's bedroom. On one wall was a set of pegs with chains and a leather whip hanging down. In the closet were two or three sequined dresses. On the dresser was a Barbie doll in a red chiffon gown and a picture of David all done up in a similar red chiffon gown. I thought right then that David's father must be sad for the son he'd never really known.

David died at 25 in 1993

Santa Claus

I don't see dead people all the time the way I used to. Well, of course part of it is the people I see who are dying – which is what I do, see people who are dying – don't look like they're dead anymore. They're not really dying as they return to work and make new plans, or they are – dying – but the time frame is all mixed up now and no one can begin to tell them when. So, the live people I see are not really dying, not anytime soon, and they certainly don't qualify as dead, even those one or two who have lost all their hair to chemotherapy and their weight to nausea and cryptosporidium and their minds to toxoplasmosis or meningitis. So that takes care of them.

But the ones I'm talking about are the dead people who have, in fact, died, one week ago or ten years ago. I used to see them everywhere – in the grocery store, on the street so I'd almost honk, coming out of a shop or a movie and almost bumping into me without the slightest hint of recognition on their faces. It made no rhyme or reason. I could see someone I barely knew seven years ago and didn't particularly like just as easily as I could bump into my dearest and fondest who had only left me weeks before.

Seeing dead people came as a type of hallucination or mistakening, but sometimes I saw people because I wanted it to be true. Nathan was someone like that, and I saw him all the time in the weeks and months after he died. He was nearly bald, not by fashion but by middle age, though no one that knew him would have guessed he was a day over thirty. He had two thick silver rings in both ears and a thin nose ring. On both arms were tattoos with vines and leaves snaking up and down. He mostly wore heavy boots, jeans, and a black leather jacket, whether or not he was riding his motorcycle with its cherry-red crankcase.

He used to work at a store on Castro Street, a little whole foods store where he was the vitamin specialist before I knew him. The irony of this never occurred to him as he'd leave the store every evening and head home for hours of snorting cocaine in the isolation of his small apartment. It never occurred to him until a counselor for a stress management program told him he was an addict. Nathan never used another drug after that, staying clean the last five years and two months of his life.

I never actually saw Nathan at the store, alive or dead, but for the longest time I'd just end up there, so I could imagine him selling vitamins, convincing people with his elfin grin and his persuasive hustle to buy things they'd never heard of.

The Nathan I would have liked to run into was the one described by a friend at his memorial service in a packed synagogue just a block from his apartment. It appears that every year in December, Nathan would go down to the main post office at Rincon Annex and ask to see the Dear Santa letters. He would spend a long time reading them and then he would pick out two or three. Somewhere out there is a little Vietnamese boy growing up in the Tenderloin who thinks Santa Claus is this bald little Jewish guy from Chicago riding a cherry-red motorcycle bringing toys.

My imaginings about Nathan had a different character from the sudden, unexpected appearances of those gone and nearly forgotten. But a few years ago, all these sightings abruptly stopped. I haven't seen a dead person in so long it probably would unnerve me if I did, even though I used to find it quite comforting. Perhaps at some metaphysical level my psyche anticipated the changing ratio of live people to dead ones that has become the epidemic. Perhaps the message is to focus, as they have done, on the living rather than on the dead.

Nathan died at 46 in 1993

PART 2

TEACHINGS

Breaking the Rules:
Psychotherapy with People with AIDS

Presented at AIDS '93: The Social Work Response: The Fifth International Conference on Social Work and AIDS: San Francisco: June 23-26, 1993

In my first meeting with my first therapy client with AIDS we talked briefly about his illness and how he was feeling. Then he looked right at me and asked, "Do you think it's okay to want to die?" I thought about it and responded, "Do you think it's okay?" Without a moment's hesitation he shot back, "Don't give me that shit, that's what my psychiatrist used to tell me."

That was in 1984. I've spent most of the last nine years working with people with AIDS in various roles, including therapist. I've learned many things from the people I've worked with, but one of the most important things I learned that day – psychotherapy with people with AIDS is different from other forms of psychotherapy. And as social workers doing this work, we often find ourselves breaking the rules of traditional psychotherapy.

Today, I want to begin to look at some of the ways this work is different – the issues clients bring to us, how we negotiate our boundaries and manage multiple roles, how transference and countertransference are affected, and how we must alter our goals and our emotional investment to fit a limited time frame.

Therapy with people with AIDS is a time-driven therapy. Before undertaking it, the therapist must examine his or her own attitudes toward working with someone who is dying. Does this work feel futile, too depressing or hopeless, like a waste of time since the person is going to die anyway? Or, does it feel like an opportunity to work with someone during a stage of life with tremendous potential for growth, helping him or her resolve all kinds of past issues, being a witness, a midwife if you will, ushering this person toward the final transition? If you're like most of us, the answer is somewhere in between. It's the initial countertransference issue to be explored before you have even met your client. It's also an issue that will resurface as the work proceeds – how to find a balance between helplessness and hopefulness.

Working with people with AIDS is not like working with people with other life-threatening illnesses. There is no cure. You know it and your clients know it, no matter how tenaciously you both may cling to your denial mechanisms. Death is a third party to every therapy session, though it may go unacknowledged for weeks or months as other issues are attended to. The existential crisis of death underlies all else that happens in the therapy. A teacher of mine, Judy Pollatsek, once said, "The true knowledge that you're going to die is like staring into the sun. You can only do it for a few seconds and then you look away. In the meantime, you're living."

I feel it is important to look at who comes for therapy. I would say that people with AIDS seeking psychotherapy fall roughly into three categories. The first category of clients are those suffering from serious mental health problems unrelated to but certainly exacerbated by their AIDS diagnosis. These clients may have psychotic, affective, or severe characterological disorders and may require psychiatric care or a day treatment program. Also in this category are those exhibiting fairly advanced stages of dementia. Although the social worker may have a case management role with these clients, he or she will probably not find psychotherapy to be useful.

A second category of clients are those who would have sought psychotherapy regardless of health status. Many people come to their AIDS diagnosis with a therapy relationship already in place or have positive previous experience in treatment and naturally seek it out during stressful times. These clients may be well served by a traditional approach to therapy, albeit an approach that allows for flexibility, as I will discuss.

There is, however, a third type of client. These are the clients who previous to AIDS were perfectly well adjusted, who have no experience with therapy, and who may have little insight or capacity to be introspective. These clients come to us because their previously adequate coping mechanisms are proving inadequate in the fact of the ultimate crisis. What they need is a supportive counseling approach that will shore up the ego strengths they have relied on throughout their lives.

In my experience, therapy with people with AIDS comes in waves, from crisis to crisis, adjustment to adjustment. There may be long periods of calm when the client inclined to introspection can make great strides toward gaining insight. These same periods of calm for a less insightful client may be a time when the therapist might suggest meeting less frequently. Intermittent supportive counseling can be increased as the need arises. When it does, clients in both categories will need a place to vent, to mourn, to refocus, and to problem-solve.

One of the ways I believe that social workers are uniquely prepared to work with people with AIDS is that we are trained in a variety of treatment modalities. AIDS demands us to be flexible, and we are able to constantly reassess our clients' needs and plan accordingly.

A few years ago, I saw a client for weekly psychotherapy for about six months. He was newly diagnosed with Kaposi's sarcoma and four years into recovery from drugs and alcohol. He talked about experiencing his feelings for the first time in his life and what a rich and exhilarating time this was for him. He was clearly engaged in the therapeutic process and was exploring issues of identity, family, sexuality, etc. Then one day he arrived with the news that he had been diagnosed with pulmonary Kaposi's sarcoma, a disease with a dismal prognosis. All of a sudden, his desire to do insight-oriented work vanished. Survival and how to maintain his quality of life were now his issues.

In my position as AIDS Project Coordinator at Jewish Family and Children's Services I wear many hats. At this time, I was about to start a short-term support group with a rabbi focusing on spiritual concerns, and I was also recruiting speakers for an education program. This client became interested in both possibilities. Although our previous contract had been to limit his involvement with the agency to therapy, his new medical situation changed both his needs and what could be seen as therapeutic for him. We terminated therapy, I referred him to a new therapist, and he became both a group member and an important contributor to the education program.

I believe this kind of flexible approach is necessary to best serve the changing needs of our clients. Flexibility may mean switching from an insight-oriented approach to a supportive counseling one, changing how frequently or infrequently we meet with a client, or, as in this case, choosing between modalities and social work interventions to find what will be the most helpful.

As therapists we need to be able to approach a client's resistance in a more open way. When this client told me one day that he didn't like the direction my questions were taking and didn't want to talk about his mother that day, it was important that I could see how the threat to his life was superseding his need to understand his intrapsychic functioning.

One of the most challenging ways that AIDS demands us to be flexible has to do with boundaries – when to cross them, what to do once we have, and how to analyze and use the insight we and our clients can gain when a boundary violation has occurred. The following example looks at how an altered therapeutic frame can alter our decisions about boundaries and also speaks to the unpredictability of this work.

One of my clients was a 27-year-old gay man who had already been diagnosed with AIDS for 3 years when I began seeing him. Although not terribly insightful, he used the therapy for support for his sobriety and it appeared to be a stabilizing influence in his life. He developed an idealized transference toward me that seemed to be a positive force, counteracting a lifetime of shame, guilt, and low self-esteem and also served to move him along in the process of taking care of himself. One of the issues we focused on was his inability to grieve. He felt emotionally shut down and yearned to be able to cry.

One day my client arrived at my office with his lover, who was in a wheelchair. The two men had met only recently and moved in together, and then the lover had taken a sharp turn for the worse. Mobility problems and dementia meant he couldn't be left alone. My client was feeling overloaded with his responsibility and with his lover's intrusion into his therapy time. Partway through the session he said, "I'm just not ready to lose him" and began to cry. If we had been alone, I'm quite sure I would have let him cry, but in this case, I went to him and gave him a hug. I remember in supervision being asked, "What made you think that hugging your client was the appropriate intervention?" and feeling angry at the insensitivity of the question. But when I analyze it, in fact I do know why. I wasn't the one who broke the boundary. The boundary was broken when my client's lover entered the room. Within that altered therapeutic frame, I was trying to recreate the holding environment my client had previously enjoyed in his sessions with me. And in our sessions following this one, it was clear that my intervention had been both significant and helpful.

I can look back on many times when I've crossed a boundary. Several times I've called a cab for a blind client, and many times I've gotten a glass of water so a client could take some pills. I once drove a man 35 miles to an AIDS clinic after spending six months of therapy focusing on his fears of seeking medical treatment. And in one case, that of the couple I've described, I responded to an emergency telephone call by going to my client's apartment to wait with him until the funeral home came to get his lover's body.

These and many other examples range in intensity and are motivated by practicality, medical urgency, and humanity. I am grounded in the human aspect of this work, but when I make a decision to act in the realm of my real relationship with my client, I am doing so consciously. I am informed by my knowledge of my clients and the expected consequences of my actions. More than that, I make sure that the therapy addresses the incident that has happened in order to explore the meaning for the client.

Sometimes we make difficult choices about setting. I generally only visit therapy clients at home once they are in a terminal phase of their illness. We all know, however, how unpredictable this disease can be and how hard it is to determine what is in fact terminal.

Last year I was working with a young man who became homebound for a month's time with Pneumocystis pneumonia and failing vision. We decided I would see him at home and I did so twice. The first visit went well, although I had to adjust to sitting on his mattress on the floor since there was nowhere else in the room to sit. On my second visit, he was again in bed, but his shirt was open and he was administering intravenous medication into a catheter in his chest. I found this distracting, to say the least, and also disturbing. I felt I was being tested in some way, and yet in the moment, felt incapable of addressing the discomfort this caused me. When my client was better and returned to my office, he was the one who brought up the fact that he had found my home visits disruptive and that maybe we should not have seen each other at all for that month.

As with so many apparent mistakes in therapy, however, this one became useful grist for the mill. It opened up a whole new arena in terms of the transference. This client felt exposed. He felt I had intruded. He felt embarrassed, unfit to be seen, judged. This was a man who had lost his mother when he was nine and who had developed a strong transference toward me involving his need for my approval, acceptance, and love. My intrusion allowed him to explore more deeply his longing for his mother and all she represented and to sort out some deep-seated feelings.

Not all shifts in setting will yield such positive effect. Often it is difficult for the therapist to maintain some sense of equilibrium and tune out distractions – IVs, urinals, half-eaten meals in the hospital, photos and objects and even sexual paraphernalia in someone's home. Maintaining the frame is not always easy. I have found a few things helpful. First, I allow myself some time to get settled and I comment on the surroundings as a bridge to more serious talk. Then I comment on how different it feels to be seeing the client at home or hospital or hospice as a way of giving him or her permission to explore what that may mean. Next, I give myself a break. Doing therapy in a hospital, even if the staff have been told not to disturb us, is never going to be the best situation. I lower my expectations, trying at least to offer some time for focused reflection. Oftentimes the client has saved up all kinds of things to tell me about his or her fears or thoughts about dying. But just as often, the client spends our time complaining about the food, the staff, or the medications. What I do for myself is let that be okay.

I've spoken a bit about the flexibility necessary to practice psychotherapy with people with AIDS and some of the ways this work challenges our ideas about boundaries and setting. I'd like to turn now to looking at some situations in which our therapeutic stance of neutrality is challenged and in which we are called upon to serve multiple roles.

If a general psychotherapy client says, "I know you think I should break up with my boyfriend" or "I know you don't think I'm smart enough to go to graduate school," responses such as, "What makes you say that?" or "How does that feel to think that's my opinion?" may lead to fruitful insights about the transference. It is not generally necessary or advisable to reveal one's true feelings on the subject, but much more important to explore how the client has projected feelings about inadequacy or powerlessness onto us and is relating to the therapist as an authority figure.

On the other hand, if a client with AIDS says, "I know you think I should stop using drugs" or "I know you think I should have safer sex," responding with a neutral question, such as "What makes you say that?" may not only be unhelpful but also ridiculous. In such cases neutrality is neither advisable nor believable. The challenge is how to use this kind of opening for direct influence in a positive way.

I believe that in therapy with people with AIDS we must take on various roles as the situation demands. Sometimes we are therapists, sometimes counselors, sometimes crisis intervention workers. Sometimes, even when not in a role such as my own where I am part therapist, part case worker and part many other things, we are still called upon to take on case management functions. Sometimes our role includes teaching and sometimes, as we will see in a minute, we end up acting as "first responder."

In cases where our views are clear, such as drug use or safer sex, one approach is that of a teacher. For example, I've had clients who have told me they are having unprotected sex, but it's okay because they only have it with other HIV-positive people. A neutral stance at this juncture could have dangerous consequences. Instead, I've chosen to inform the client that the current understanding of transmission is that reinfection with HIV can bring on symptoms more quickly for both parties.

We must be careful, when we give information, not to cross the line of being judgmental. Changing sexual behavior is clearly a difficult and slow process, and we must be there along the way as our clients struggle with their ambivalence, their responsibility, and their self-destructiveness.

I have a female case management client who was in therapy with someone else. She was struggling with whether she should inform her partners that she was infected and thus risk losing them – a familiar pattern for her – or delay telling them until the relationship was more stable, while practicing safer sex. Her therapist gave her an ultimatum: "Either you tell all potential sex partners that you are infected or I will no longer be able to see you in therapy." Predictably, this therapist lost her client, who was furious and quite devasted by the loss.

I believe our approach must be somewhere between ultimatums and neutral indifference. In my experience, clients who have developed a positive or idealized transference toward me have been able to borrow my superego, if you will, to change dangerous sex and drug patterns and to seek appropriate medical care. In fact, I believe the relationship has been crucial in allowing these clients to make changes, whereas direct influence by other professionals has sometimes not worked.

I've been working with an HIV-positive client for the last ten months in therapy who is addicted to IV crystal methedrine, although not to the point where he has suffered severe negative consequences. Although his immune system was showing signs of deterioration, he has been impervious to his doctor's prescription to stop using. Very slowly, however, he has been using the therapy to enter recovery, although not in the more traditional sense. He is highly resistant to 12-step approaches and has rejected all other drug treatment programs. He is not fully ready to be clean but, through the therapy, he has had longer and longer periods of abstinence and has been able to explore at length his ambivalence, his self-destructiveness, the meaning for him of sobriety, and his fears of abandoning substances that allow him to avoid his fears of HIV.

Many clinicians, in fact most, do not treat people who are still actively abusing drugs or alcohol. Yet AIDS has pushed me and many others to stretch ourselves to work with clients in early recovery, fearing the consequences to their health and that of others if we abandon them. What I've found is that providing a holding environment for the ambivalence, a place where I do not judge, but still hold on to my bias for abstinence, has allowed clients, like the one I just described, a valuable piece of pre-recovery therapy. After some early sessions with this client where I felt drawn in to being the adversary, my client was able to internalize me. He would approach the topic with, "I know how you feel about this" and later with, "I think you were right." A little bit of the teacher approach early on, pointing to physical and emotional consequences of drug use, went a long way later as he struggled with abstinence.

I should add that this client has recently taken a break from therapy. Without ever giving an ultimatum, I had discussed with him the idea that therapy would not be fully effective as long as he was still using drugs. Several months later, after a relapse, he repeated my words and said he now agreed. He is ready to take some more serious steps toward abstinence and would like to return to therapy after he has been clean and sober for 90 days. I am hopeful and quite confident that he will.

Another area where a teaching approach can be helpful is with the client who begins to show signs of dementia. Initially a client may complain of forgetting things or getting confused. I feel it's important not to minimize this experience the way friends may be doing with statements such as, "Don't worry, everybody forgets things." Dementia, next to blindness, is what most people with AIDS are most afraid of. Rather than minimize, I try to normalize the experience and teach some helpful strategies.

For example, I may say, "You know, this could have something to do with HIV in the brain, but it might also be a side effect of all the medications you're on. It could be a result of the insomnia you're reporting or it could be a natural reaction to stress." I may introduce some simple techniques to assist memory, such as using a calendar, writing lists, or taping notes on the refrigerator. And I try to explore further the person's fears about dementia. It seems obvious to say that a missed appointment by a person with AIDS may have more to do with early signs of dementia than it does with resistance to treatment, and we should be alert to this so we can make appropriate medical referrals.

Sometimes making the appropriate referrals can be of utmost importance. Our social work training allows us to respond to crises in ways many other clinicians may not feel comfortable doing. I was seeing a client with some early signs of dementia a few years ago who had taken a turn for the worse. On a home visit which was intended as a therapy session, I found that he had become completely delusional. He was lying in his own excrement and warned me not to let the snake who had been terrorizing him back into the room. In this situation, I was a "first responder" and needed to act as swiftly as a paramedic. I was also terrified and overwhelmed by this responsibility that had been thrust upon me. Luckily, my familiarity with the resources in the city allowed me to quickly obtain medical and nursing backup and to start the process for getting my client into a

24-hour care facility. It's situations like these where our natural instincts and clear thinking are more important than our training as clinicians.

One of the toughest issues both emotionally and ethically that we face as clinicians is that of suicide. Over the years working with individuals and groups, the issue of suicide has come up often. My belief is that thoughts about suicide by people with AIDS are most often related to control and quality of life concerns, and that if hope and control can be enhanced or restored, the desire to die will subside.

A client of mine in his late 40s had been the last member to join an ongoing support group I ran for a year and a half. A few months after the group had ended, he asked if I could come to see him, and when I did, he told me he had decided to commit suicide. He was in a lot of pain and his medical situation was deteriorating rapidly. He had spoken with his sister, his lover, and his doctor, and all had agreed that this was a rational and dignified plan. Now he wanted me to find a rabbi for him to talk with as well. I arranged this and then waited to hear that he'd carried out his plan. As the days and then weeks progressed, I began to suspect that he really wouldn't kill himself. In fact, he lived a full year after our conversation and died of natural complications of AIDS.

Several months later, I received a call from another man, who I'd seen intermittently for counseling at crisis points in his illness. He was now homebound and on oxygen and when I went to see him, he also wanted to talk about suicide. My approach to him showed a willingness to talk about the issue, but did not hide my bias. It brought in an element of teaching and also something I call "bringing the support group into the room."

I spoke to him about how much ambivalence goes into making the decision to commit suicide, and I told him that my role is to be on the side of life in helping him explore his ambivalence. We reviewed different aspects of his life that still brought him joy and discussed ways he might minimize the pain of some other aspects. And then I told him the story of the first man. I told him that in the year he had lived after he had decided to die there had been several days when he was well enough to walk down the block and sit in the sun in the park and how much he had enjoyed the company of his old friends who made special trips to visit him that last year. By using the stories of clients whom we have worked with, while protecting their anonymity, we can expand the realm of our clients' experience. In this case, my client seemed relieved, and our talk in the upcoming months focused more on living than on dying.

In closing, I'd like to tell one more story from my experience, one that exemplifies my belief that clients are the ones who really know what they need. If we can open ourselves, if we can really listen, they will tell us what it is they need.

I met this client when he was 23. He used a variety of the services of our program, and when he was 25, he started therapy with me. During the next year he lost much of his vision, took a break from therapy to travel to New Zealand, Australia, and his native England, returned to San Francisco, lost the rest of his vision, and made a miraculous adjustment to his blindness. One day he came to my office looking dishelved and walking in an uncoordinated fashion. He had a hard time staying awake, so finally I asked, "What is it that you would want from me know?" He said, "I just want you to sit by my bed while I go to sleep." A few days later he entered the hospital with a lung infection and while there suffered a series of seizures. In the next few weeks I visited him several times in the hospital and then in a nursing home, reminiscing with him about his life, though he could barely speak, stroking his hair, and just being there, sitting by his bed while he went to sleep.

If there's one belief I hold most strongly about working with people with AIDS, it is that we need to be prepared to go the distance with them. I have been profoundly privileged to be able to work with people living and dying with AIDS, to be a therapist, a witness, a midwife. I urge you, too, to embrace this work and know that the rewards far outweigh the many, many losses.

Chaplaincy Training

Presented as an in-service training for the Clinical Pastoral Training Program at Mt. Zion Hospital in San Francisco, 1996

A client of mine, whom I'll call Jonathan, told me this story. In 1983 he was living in Oklahoma working as an attorney for a gas and oil company. His partner of many years, a research physician, had died six months earlier of what was still being called Gay Related Immune Deficiency. When Jonathan himself was hospitalized with Pneumocystis pneumonia and given a diagnosis of AIDS he was also given a prognosis of less than six months to live. He did what many people would have done – he called his clergy person, in this case the rabbi he'd known since he moved to Oklahoma.

The rabbi arrived at the hospital, but when he realized the diagnosis, he began a tirade: "How could you have brought me here and endangered my life?" It would have been bad enough if the rabbi had rejected the *mitzvot*, or commandment, to visit the sick and given in to his own fears of transmission. But this rabbi went further. Although he had known that Jonathan was gay and had met his late partner, he now castigated him for his homosexuality and blamed him for bringing the disease on himself.

There is a hopeful note to this ghastly story and that is that Jonathan stood fast to his faith. "That was just one bad rabbi, and I wasn't going to let one bad rabbi take away my Judaism."

Thankfully, few of the people we work with have had to withstand the kind of abuse Jonathan suffered when he was most in need, most actively reaching out to his religious tradition for guidance. And yet, there are echoes of his story in many of the stories I've heard in the 13 years I've been working with people with AIDS.

Homophobia is so deeply ingrained in our Judeo-Christian frame of reference that no gay person in our society can escape stigmatization. At one level there is the prejudice, discrimination, and outright hatred often displayed toward gay people. Parents disown their children, great rifts open up between siblings, silence descends, fathers sit *shivah* for their sons.

But perhaps more destructive than the outward rejection is the toll internalized homophobia takes. The most common story I've heard in the past seven years from clients at Jewish Family and Children's Services has been: "Sometime around my bar mitzvah, when I realized I was gay, I realized there was no place for me in the Jewish community, so I turned away." In the years I worked in a nonsectarian environment, this same thinking translated more often into: "I knew I wasn't following the teachings of the church," or "I knew I'd be damned in hell." These are harsh messages for an adult to endure, yet alone a boy of 13.

At an even deeper level, the negative messages many people with AIDS have received have been integrated into their images of themselves. For those who grow up in supportive families and communities and find ways to continue to practice their religion, that outcome is the best. There is nothing like professional and economic success, good relationships, and a well-rounded social life to counteract early messages that being gay is bad, sinful, and shameful. But there are many others for whom the "wrongness" of homosexuality becomes inextricably linked to all the other failures in one's life. I rarely hear a successful client bemoan the fact that he is gay, even though he would perhaps be AIDS-free if he were heterosexual. But for those individuals who feel themselves to have failed in one or more aspects of their lives, being gay sometimes becomes the culprit.

In 1984 I was leading a support group in Washington, D.C. that was large and religiously and ethnically mixed. Partway through a session one of the members said, "I feel that AIDS was a gift from God so I can atone for my sins." Although this caused quite an uproar, with another member jumping from his chair and yelling, "What do you mean, 'sins'?" I believe the power of internalized homophobia was informing this young man's sense of self.

This is where ministry, chaplaincy, pastoral care can be most useful. The late Father Bill Wendt, whom I had the pleasure of working with at the St. Francis Center in Washington, D.C., used to call working with dying patients "a ministry of presence." As a social worker I know how important "being with" can be, particularly when a client is terminal. But I also know that what people often need is some connection to their faith tradition, to an important aspect of their formative years by which they may no longer feel embraced. Certainly there are elements of prayer and ritual, atonement and preparation for death, all of which we'll be talking about, but at the most basic level, people want to be accepted back into the fold. A visit from a priest or a rabbi or a minister to a patient who feels unworthy can be of ultimate value in the healing process.

Before we leave the topic of stigma, I'd like to mention that although 70% of new cases of AIDS in San Francisco are still being seen in gay or bisexual men, they do not have a corner of the market on stigma. Women, often overlooked by the medical system as potential HIV patients because they are seen as "nice girls," often suffer terribly when they are diagnosed and are subject to external or internal messages that they aren't quite as "nice" as they thought they were. Other women, supporting themselves, their children, and their drug habits through prostitution are so rejected by our society that they give up expecting a religious person to take notice of them.

There is a common misperception about substance abusers, who make up the fastest-growing group of people with AIDS, and that is that they have no conscience. What I have found is that they often have the opposite – an overblown sense of superego, conscience, and guilt. They also tend to have poor self-esteem, although it is sometimes buried under a load of narcissistic bravado. Pastoral care is often the last thing a substance abuser thinks he or she deserves, and yet attention to spirituality has everything to do with recovery.

A few years ago, I was working with a heroin addict in his early thirties. After two incarcerations in state prison and two bouts of Pneumocystis pneumonia, he came in for a session looking a little guilty. "I went to this barbecue this weekend put on by one of the big AIDS organizations. I thought I was eating beef ribs, they were really good, but they turned out to be pork ribs. I've never eaten pork my whole life." Here was a young man, slamming heroin into his veins every day and suffering from AIDS, who had somehow found meaning behind keeping the basic dietary laws of his religion. These moments, these windows give those of us in the helping professions an opening for healing.

In my early years of AIDS work, most of the focus on ritual came around planning for funerals and memorial services. In 1983, people with AIDS were dying in a matter of weeks or months. Even when I left the D.C. area at the end of 1989, the average longevity for an African-American man with AIDS was only nine months from diagnosis and less for a woman. So ritual was important for survivors, even when it was not able to be a tool of healing incorporated into the everyday life of the person with AIDS. One of the things that was so striking to see was how intricately people, given the chance, would plan their own sendoffs.

The first person with AIDS I worked with, as a volunteer, was a 40-year-old man who owned a bicycle shop. He lived with his partner and had custody of his teenage son and daughter. He survived a full year after diagnosis. His Presbyterian funeral was very formal, and his partner's name or existence was never mentioned. But at the end, per his instructions, three clowns came down the aisles and gave everyone balloons. Then we went outside and were supposed to let go of the balloons. I still remember how hard it was for his daughter to let go.

In 1984 the Morticians' Union in New York State went on strike, saying they would not handle the bodies of people who had died of AIDS. This and other aspects of AIDS hysteria caused many people with AIDS to choose cremation when they might not otherwise have done so.

I remember Jesse, another person I volunteered for, saying to me in his crass, sarcastic way, "I'm not sure how I'm going to tell my parents I want to be burned instead of planted." The way he chose was to include many other traditions from his Tennessee Methodist upbringing. His service included a fancy memorial bulletin with his picture and a recording of him addressing the audience. The next week an urn with his ashes was buried on his land in Tennessee and a pink dogwood, the symbol of the resurrection because of red at the tips of the flowers, was planted. He had planned it all, even the menu for the reception following at a friend's house. I remember the last time I saw him I asked how long he felt he might live. He replied, "Well, I have to live until Tuesday, because that's when my next SSI check is coming and I need it to pay for the funeral."

I certainly would not want to see the role of a chaplain be diminished to simply funeral planning. And yet I see the significance for many people of being able to "plan for their own immortality." Oftentimes we are working with young people – Jesse was 29 when he died – who may not have had a chance to accomplish what they may have wished. A fancy or elaborate or outrageous memorial service may be an opportunity to make a statement and to try to control how others will grieve and remember.

When I returned to San Francisco after many years in Washington and Maryland, I left many clients I'd been working with through an AIDS program at the Department of Social Services. One of them was Sheldon. He was African-American and had gone blind from AIDS. He lived in a one-bedroom apartment with his parents and his brother, a heroin addict. The electricity had been turned off, but a kind superintendent allowed them to string an extension cord into the laundry room to get some power. Sheldon was very sad when I went to say goodbye to him. He said, "Have someone put a carnation on my coffin, I'll know it's from you." That sense that cognition continues past death is not a belief I would want to tamper with.

Sometimes clients have specific questions about religious practices and are only satisfied if they can ask a clergy person. In Judaism there is a probation against desecration of the body. No one with a tattoo, for instance, is allowed to be buried in an Orthodox cemetery. Several years ago, a client of mine with a tattoo was planning to be buried in an Orthodox cemetery in his home state and was in a terrible quandary. It was important that he had a chance to speak with a rabbi, who explained the side of the religion that allows for compassion even when a rule has been broken.

Compassion was also what guided the community of a Carmelite monk who attended my support group in 1985. Each week a different monk from the monastery would bring him to group and wait to bring him home. When he became ill the brothers cared for him within the monastery, and his mother and sister were with him when he died.

I'd like to turn to one of the most powerful experiences I've had in the past seven years at Jewish Family and Children's Services, which has been cofacilitating a "spiritual support group" with Rabbi Nancy Flam, who in 1991 founded the Bay Area Jewish Healing Center. The group, for six men and one woman with AIDS, was designed to allow members to explore their Jewish identities and to see what Judaism had to offer in times of illness. The participants, for the most part, were so estranged and distanced from their Judaism that one was even surprised to learn that women were now being ordained in the Reform movement.

Through eight weeks of readings and teachings, questioning and prayer, this group individually and collectively returned to their Jewish roots. They formed strong bonds with each other. The member who had been a practicing Buddhist for 25 years discovered that, "It was always here in my own backyard, in my own tradition." When the group ended, three of the members bought each other yarmulkes, had Passover seder together, began attending Shabbat services and healing services, and eventually joined the synagogue – as a family.

A part of AIDS that is always present is grief. Not only do people with AIDS lose health, productivity, livelihood, potency, ability to plan for the future, ad infinitum, most people with AIDS living today have lost many of their friends, partners, and family members to the illness. One area where ritual can be most effective is creating a space to grieve. Allowing people with AIDS to use the rituals of their traditions allows them to separate each loss, honor each loss and move on, rather than suffering from an overwhelming cumulative state of grief. Whether reciting *Kaddish* on the anniversary of a death, lighting a candle and saying a blessing, or creating a panel for the Names Memorial Quilt, clients can find comfort.

Prayers are said for the dead, but they are also said for the living. Whether or not a faith tradition has a specific prayer for healing in its liturgy, one can be introduced. Saying prayers that give blessing and praise, reciting the Psalms, practicing Zen or other forms of meditation – all can be healing. In my support group for people with HIV/AIDS who are substance abusers and who are interested in exploring their Jewish identities, someone suggested writing a gratitude list, which is a tool from Alcoholics Anonymous. Each day one writes down five things to be grateful for. Someone else in the group mentioned that this is similar to reciting the *Modeh Ani*, the Jewish morning blessing.

When I started working with people with AIDS, I thought there would be a lot of moments of true awe, of amazing connection, of love and excruciating loss. I thought there would be great existential moments that I would witness. I remember one. A client said, "I feel the pull of the universe on me." But much of the work is about arguments between roommates, unresolved family issues, diarrhea, depression, Social Security applications. It's not always interesting and it's not always pretty.

And not every client is lovable. In fact, when people ask me, "How can you do this work?" I often say, "Thank God I don't fall in love with all of them." And yet, as Father Bill Wendt and his ministry of presence used to say, "You must be free to fall in love."

I am aware that I've been speaking about AIDS in the context of death and dying today and yet HIV and AIDS are changing so rapidly that everything we've known is up for question. My hope, of course, is that AIDS will become a chronic, manageable illness and that people with HIV will look to religion for more than just an answer about cremation versus burial. But I also know that people will continue to die of AIDS for a long time and that their only contacts with religion or spirituality might be from you, their chaplains in a hospital. And so, I'm glad to have been here today and I'm happy to answer any of your questions.

Providing Jewish AIDS Services: Making the Case for Culturally Specific Programming

Keynote address, International Jewish AIDS Network Conference, Washington, DC, October 10, 1996

By 1985, 2,035 people in San Francisco had been diagnosed with AIDS. Approximately 100 were Jewish. But when Jewish Family and Children's Services of San Francisco, the Peninsula, Marin and Sonoma Counties applied for a grant from the Endowment Fund of the Jewish Community Federation, they were turned down. AIDS was not a Jewish issue.

In 1986, another 1,388 San Franciscans were diagnosed with AIDS, bringing the total number of Jewish people with AIDS in the City to about 170. The Jewish Community Endowment Newhouse Fund reversed its position and came through with a grant, which has been renewed each year, providing partial funding for the AIDS Family Outreach Project, now known simply as the AIDS Project.

Not all programs around the country that have sought to establish AIDS services have had an easy time of answering that fundamental question: Is AIDS a Jewish issue? Some of you here today and many who would have wanted to be here are struggling with boards and administrations reluctant to allocate funds, serve stigmatized populations, or provide lifesaving services for our youth.

Today I'd like to go beyond the question of whether AIDS is a Jewish issue, because it seems so obvious. We, as human beings, as a light unto the nations, must serve those who are ill and in need. But how we do this is as varied as we as service providers are varied. Two main distinctions can be made – those Jewish agencies, organizations, and synagogues serving the nonsectarian AIDS community and those serving only Jewish clients.

Today I'm going to talk about the latter situation, since the program I have coordinated for the past seven years falls in this category. We serve Jewish individuals, couples, and families where one or more members are HIV-infected. In looking at what we do, I would like to move on to a different set of questions. How can Judaism be helpful in times of illness? What are the tools of our tradition that can bring strength and hope and comfort to those with AIDS? And how can culturally specific programming provide a way for our clients to claim or re-claim a vital link to their heritage?

One of the questions I get asked often is, "How do clients find you?" About six years ago, a couple from a small town in Florida wrote to Jewish Family and Children's Services in San Francisco. "Our son David lives in San Francisco and he has AIDS. We don't know where to turn. We remember that when David was a little boy, we brought him to Jewish Family Services in New Jersey, where we were living at the time. Do you think you might be able to help him?" These parents didn't know whether JFCS had an AIDS program, but they did know that Jewish Family Services has a long history of providing help to those in need in the Jewish community. In fact, San Francisco's JFCS, originally known as the Eureka Benevolent Society when it was established in 1850, is the oldest charitable institution west of the Mississippi.

In this case I called the couple and set up an appointment for when they would be visiting and encouraged them to bring their son, which they did. I worked with him to get him on disability, to find AIDS housing, and to set him up with our meal delivery program, the Chicken Soupers. I also saw him for weekly therapy for the last year and a half of his life.

I have often been frustrated to hear a social worker from a hospital or another agency say, "I was working with a person with AIDS who was Jewish, but I didn't refer him to you because he didn't go to synagogue." In a region known for its high rate of assimilation – only 15% of the quarter million Jews in the San Francisco Bay Area are affiliated with a synagogue – it is sometimes difficult to explain to non-Jews and Jews alike all the facets that make up one's Jewish identity. One way to address this lack of understanding is to provide in-service trainings for the staff of other agencies. When I do this, I am not only describing our services but also speaking about what it means to be a Jew. This allows other service providers to better identify who should be referred to our program.

I'd like to talk about some of the ways that clients of the AIDS Project have found to express their Jewish connection through using our services. Whether the connection is religious, Zionist, a memory of grandmother's cooking, or a haunting identification with victims or survivors of the Holocaust, there are feelings to be explored. So, in addition to providing high quality social services, volunteer opportunities, and educational outreach, the AIDS Project has a commitment to nurturing Jewish identity.

This is especially important when you consider whom we serve. The demographics of AIDS in San Francisco are unlike anywhere in the world. 81.6% of cases reported through March of 1996 were in gay and bisexual men, with an additional 9.2% of cases in gay and bisexual men who are also injection drug users. That's a total of 90.8% of all cases in San Francisco, whereas nationwide for new cases in 1995, only 42% were in men who have sex with men. The percentage for those served by the AIDS

Project (approximately 100 every year) is similar – 90 to 95% are gay or bisexual men.

When I first meet with a new client, I conduct an intake interview, usually lasting about an hour and a half. I ask about the person's medical history, living and financial situation, the work he or she did or is doing, support from partner or family, psychiatric and substance abuse history if any, and, last but not least, Jewish connection. The most common story I hear when a client is a gay man, whether he was raised Orthodox, Conservative, or Reform, is, "soon after my bar mitzvah I realized I was gay and that there was no place for me in the Jewish community." It is small wonder that gay Jewish men from Brooklyn to Baltimore, from South Bend, Indiana to Mobile, Alabama come to San Francisco, the gay Mecca, and end up submerging and ignoring their Judaism.

Including a question about Jewish identity right at the beginning of the helping relationship opens a possibility for dialogue. Sometimes it leads to requests for referrals, such as a synagogue, where to buy a yahrzeit candle, or how to find a good bagel. And sometimes it becomes a theme that will be reexplored in therapy or support group. Allowing a client to talk about who he or she is, vis-à-vis Jewish identity, is something unique that we can offer as a Jewish agency.

Obviously, not all of our clients are interested in connecting with their Jewish roots. Some of them come for financial assistance, playing the Jewish card most to their advantage. Others come for our variety of support and volunteer services – case management, psychotherapy, support groups for people with AIDS and their families, meal delivery, "practical support" volunteers, or the possibility of serving on our speakers' bureau for the "Putting a Face to AIDS" education program. And yet walking through our door instead of one of the doors of another AIDS organization in San Francisco signals some acknowledgment. They may not

72

know that our services are delivered with a Jewish flavor and an understanding or Jewish identity issues, but something feels right about coming to us.

Paul Monette, an early AIDS author and poet, wrote, "War is not all death it turns out war is what little thing you hold on to refugeed and far from home." I think of that line when I think of a client who was fighting the demons of heroin addiction. One day he came in to see me looking a little guilty and admitted he'd accidentally eaten pork at an AIDS organization event. "I've never eaten pork my whole life," he said. Here was a young man slamming heroin into his veins every day and suffering from AIDS who had somehow found meaning behind keeping the basic laws of *kashrut*. The fact that I could hear that and not minimize its meaning points to the special nature of culturally sensitive services.

I remember a client I saw in therapy for two years. After high school he had stayed in his small Northern California community for quite some time working odd jobs and teaching Hebrew school at the local Conservative synagogue. When he came to San Francisco he made a break from Judaism, blaming it for keeping him from coming out as who he really was. He seemed to have nothing but disdain for his Jewish background. And then one day he asked me where I was going for my upcoming vacation. After doing the usual therapist's routine of exploring what it meant to him, I told him I was going to Israel. He didn't seem to react much, but as he walked out of my office he turned and said, "Put my name in the Wailing Wall and say a prayer for me."

Sometimes clients come specifically for a Jewish environment. I was interviewing a client named Jonathan for a support group I was about to start. He told me an awful story about being mistreated by a rabbi who blamed him for his illness and for putting the rabbi at risk by calling him to his bedside. Jonathan, by this point a long-term survivor, was able to say, "He was just one bad rabbi, and I wasn't going to let one bad rabbi take away my Judaism." To the contrary, he was seeking out a Jewish support group. "I want a group where I can say I just spent $5,000 on my funeral arrangements and not have someone say, 'You should get cremated, it's so much cheaper'."

Jonathan found such a group at the AIDS Project. It met for a year and a half. When one of the members who had joined a few months before converting to Judaism went to the *mikvah*, he asked Jonathan to be his witness.

San Francisco is a city that prides itself on multiculturalism in service delivery. There is the African-American AIDS Project, the Black AIDS Coalition, the Filipino AIDS Project, Instituto Familiar de la Raza, the Asian-Pacific Islander AIDS Coalition, and not one, but two programs serving Native Americans with AIDS. And yet, when it comes to Jews, the need for culturally specific programs has not always been recognized by agencies or by the clients themselves. Some aren't aware that it might feel more comfortable and familiar to sit in a room with other Jews until they have done so.

My most recent support group was an eight-week session for those with asymptomatic HIV. It was a small group of high-functioning men – a doctor, a computer programmer, a designer, a hospital administrator, and a clinical psychologist. In the first session they seemed to be falling over backwards to convince each other that being Jewish didn't mean much to them. One came from a "completely secular home," another was a "red diaper baby," a term in and of itself most often associated with Jews. And yet as the weeks passed there was an occasional comment about how nice it was to be with other Jews. Certain terminology would creep in – "So what am I, chopped liver?" And on the seventh session, one of the members initiated a lengthy discussion about what the upcoming High Holidays meant to everyone.

The AIDS Project does not act in a vacuum. Our Chicken Souper meal program is a program we coordinate but which is run by Conservative Congregation Beth Sholom and Reform Congregation Sherith Israel. Our Practical Support volunteers come in all ages and from all walks of life. Synagogues and singles groups, third grade classes, and adult education courses give us their *tzedakah* money or deliver special baskets for Hanukkah, Passover, and Rosh Hashanah. Synagogues all over the city, but especially Congregation Sha'ar Zahav, the predominantly gay and lesbian synagogue, give free tickets for High Holidays and Passover. And the Jewish Film Festival, which some think of as our largest Jewish festival, gives free passes to all our clients for all showings each year.

Leslie is someone for whom the holidays mean a lot. Raised in an upper-middle-class home in Philadelphia, she fell on hard times, and ended up a prostitute and cocaine addict. She became pregnant by her long-term boyfriend, also a person with AIDS. But she continued to use cocaine throughout her pregnancy, and the baby was born dead. A Jewish woman doctor at San Francisco General Hospital connected her up with the Jewish Mortuary so Leslie could give her baby a Jewish burial. By doing so she also reestablished her ties to Judaism. Leslie has been clean and sober for three years; her boyfriend is currently in an inpatient treatment program. And for the last three years, they've been able to attend both High Holiday services and the Congregational Seder at Congregation Sha'ar Zahav.

Leslie has recently asked for my help. She and her boyfriend have now been together for ten years, somehow surviving the horrors of drug addiction and stillbirth. When he finishes his drug treatment program, they would like to get married. But since they both depend on Supplemental Security Income, marriage would lower their income significantly. "Do you think you could find us a rabbi that would perform a Jewish wedding without the civil part?" she asked me. I've already found someone.

Leslie isn't the only one with marriage on her mind. A client named Ben, who is bedridden, and his non-Jewish partner of seven years had hoped to get married in Hawaii, if it legalizes gay marriages. But with time running out for Ben, they decided to have a commitment ceremony instead and asked that I find a rabbi. I did, through the Bay Area Jewish Healing Center. She not only performed a lovely ceremony, but has now been providing regular pastoral counseling for Ben.

One of the most powerful experiences I've had in the past seven years has been co-facilitating a "spiritual support group" with Rabbi Nancy Flam, who in 1991 founded the Bay Area Jewish Healing Center. Through eight weeks of readings and teachings, questioning and prayer, this group individually and collectively returned to its Jewish roots. They formed strong bonds with each other. When the group ended, three of the members bought each other *yarmulkes*, had Passover seder together, began attending Shabbat services and healing services, and eventually joined a synagogue together – as a family.

One of the three, Nathan, a recovering drug addict in his mid-40s, went on to become a hardworking member both of our speakers' bureau and our advisory committee, along with numerous other volunteer endeavors. In the spring of 1993, he decided he wanted to visit Israel for the first time and planned to do so with a congregational trip. The problem was he had no money. Never one to be stopped by something so simple, Nathan wrote a letter to every rabbi in Northern California telling them of his plight. Within weeks, Hebrew school children were raising money, some with creative campaigns, such as "Buy Nathan a cab ride in Tel Aviv, Buy Nathan a falafel in Jerusalem."

Sadly, Nathan never made it to Israel. He died about a month before the trip. But as he lay in the hospital on a respirator, he was aware that more donations had arrived, meeting his goal. The Jewish community had reached out to him to help him fulfill his dream.

The story doesn't end there. After Nathan's death, donations were returned and donors were given the option to send money to other AIDS causes or to a fund to send another Jew with AIDS on a first-time visit to Israel. A small fund was set up and two year later another AIDS Project client, Jeff, was given a grant.

Jeff had not known Nathan directly, but he knew who he was. He asked for a picture of him. When he returned from his trip, he told me how he had walked the streets of the Old City, taking Nathan on a guided tour in his mind. When he came to the Wailing Wall, it was time to let him go. "I know it set the universe right," he said, "but it was sad. By the time I took him to the Wall, I had developed this emotional bond with him. But in a sense, he made it to Israel finally."

Each year the AIDS Project serves one or two clients from Israel. There is no question that they feel more comfortable at a Jewish agency. A few months ago, the parents of one of my Israel clients were visiting. This young man had only tested positive six or seven months before and also had a low T-cell count. He had not wanted to tell his parents in Haifa over the phone. So, he waited for their visit and the day after telling them brought them in to see me to help them deal with the shock. I was able to listen, offer comfort, and assure them that our program would provide as many resources as possible for their son, including connecting him to other programs in the city.

For some clients the connection to Judaism is related to the Holocaust. Several clients have had parents who were survivors and one older gentleman had been a child survivor himself. I remember speaking with a mother, her concentration camp number exposed on her forearm, while her son, a prominent immigration attorney, lay in a coma in the next room.

The identification with the Holocaust is expressed in various ways. One patient in hospice had as a dying wish the desire to see the Museum of Tolerance in Los Angeles. One client willed his most cherished possession – his grandfather's concentration camp uniform – to the Holocaust Museum here in Washington.

In a group I led last summer, a member posed the question, "So, how do you keep going?" One very ill member held up his hand like this, "Five minutes, if I can just have five good minutes each day, then I'm okay." Another said, "We're Jews. We persevere." And another said, "I've been thinking a lot lately about people in concentration camps and how they survived day to day."

All these seeds, all these memory traces, all these points of connection are there.

They are there waiting for us to help rekindle a lost flame or keep one burning that may be faltering. We can start by asking the people we serve what it is in Jewish tradition that has meaning for them. We can encourage open discussion in counseling and in support groups. We can make ourselves available to a family member who might not feel comfortable at a generic AIDS organization, but would trust a Jewish agency. We can work to unlock hidden spiritual pathways. We can exalt with our clients at their newfound joy at returning to tradition. We can be part of *re'fuat hanefesh*, a healing of the body and a healing of the spirit.

And when the time comes for death, we can be there for comfort.

Sometimes it isn't clear that a client feels much connection to Judaism until after he or she has died. Robert was such a person. He was 23 when he came to the agency and 26 when he died. In keeping with the way he had lived his life, his memorial service was held in a sex club. We looked at pictures of him bald and naked posing in a graveyard. We saw a video of him camping it up in drag. We listened to a recording of him chanting in Hebrew at his *bar mitzvah*. We told wonderful, funny stories about him. And in the quiet candlelit glow of that room, 35 of us rose to say *Kaddish* for him.

For me, what has been the most precious part of working with people with AIDS has been the possibility of human connection, the possibility to truly give of myself as a human being. Working with people with AIDS in a Jewish setting has allowed me to incorporate my own renewed and evolving sense of Judaism into the work that I do. I can offer myself in a human way *and* a Jewish way.

I'd like to close with two thank-you notes I received this year. I always say I don't live for the thanks, but they're always wonderful to receive.

From a mother: "Now that *Shivah* is over, I want to get to the things that are close to my heart. This includes your beautiful chanting of *El Moleh Rachamim* at Samuel's funeral service. It came from the heart and Ernest and I will always treasure your participation at a time which will live with us to the end of our lives. I hope you will remember Samuel with a smile – he would have liked that."

And from a partner of one of the deceased: "Thank you for all that you did to provide help and assistance to Bill and me prior to his death. Your many loving acts of kindness were very much appreciated. You have dedicated yourself to a *very* worthwhile and wonderful program, which demonstrates all that is good in Judaism."

On Grief

Sermon Delivered at Congregation Sha'ar Zahav, San Francisco, December 18, 1992

When I was a teenager, I saw a movie called Harold and Maude. Perhaps some of you saw it. I saw it eight times. In the movie Harold, who's about 20, and Maude, who's almost 80 keep meeting at funerals for people neither of them have met. They get to know each other and fall in love, and they embark on a quirky eccentric love affair. On her 80th birthday Maude takes an overdose of sleeping pills as she's planned to do for a long time. When Harold finds her, he's devastated and outraged. He yells at her, "But I love you, Maude." And she replies, very calmly, "That's wonderful, now go out and love some more."

Tonight, I'm going to speak about grief and the process of mourning, about how Jewish tradition can help us with that process, and about how we can find the strength to go out and love some more.

Now you may be thinking this seems like a very dark topic to speak of as we enter our festival of lights, but we are reminded that *Adonai* created both the darkness and the light. It is our acknowledgment of and our respect for the dark that can help us to experience the light in our lives.

Hannah Senesh wrote:

"There are stars whose light reaches the earth only after they themselves have disintegrated and are no more. And there are men
[and women] whose scintillating memories light the world after they

have passed from it. These lights which shine in the darkest night
are those which illuminate for us the path."

Several years ago, before HIV antibody testing, I met a man I'll call Stan. His lover had died of AIDS just 10 days after he was diagnosed. No one at Stan's job knew that he was gay and had a lover, or that his lover had died of AIDS. So Stan went to work and cried silently in his cubicle all day. One day at noon, he ran home and ran up three flights of stairs. It wasn't until he had his key in the lock that he realized that his lover wasn't going to be there to meet him for lunch as had been their daily custom.

Surely the first, and a recurring, part of grief is denial. The process of mourning can only begin when we can acknowledge our loss. How much easier it might have been for Stan if he had been given the opportunity to talk openly about his loss and express his grief, and in so doing receive the support of his community.

Judaism in its wisdom offers us ways to break through our denial so we are not struck unaware by the empty apartment at lunchtime, the shock that someone has indeed died. We are taught not to embalm our dead and make them up to look better in death than they did in life. We bury our dead quickly and simply. We shovel dirt on their coffins, we rend our clothing, we observe the mourning period of *shivah.* These rituals make death real for us, force us to acknowledge our loss, and allow our community to support us and grieve with us.

Now you may be thinking, "What good are these rituals to me? My friend's body was sent home for burial and I couldn't be there. My lover was cremated; there was no coffin to shovel dirt on. I can't observe *shivah*, I have to go back to work. Besides, if I sat *shivah* for every person I've lost, that's all I'd ever do. Anyway, I didn't really know him that well."

Judaism has given us a ritual that can be ours to use for all our losses, individual and collective, close and not so close, recent and deep in the past.

It is the mourner's *Kaddish*, the ancient Aramaic prayer we recite as an exuberant reaffirmation of our faith in God at a time when that faith has been most severely tested. Traditionally the *Kaddish* was recited only by men in the presence of a *minyan* (a quorum of worshippers) every day. It was recited for 11 months following the death of a parent, child, sibling, or spouse. As the mourners stood, the rest of the congregation remained silent, adding "amen" at the end of each line. The mourners were thus acknowledged as separate, together forming the bond sought for in modern-day bereavement groups. At the same time, they were supported by the community as a whole.

Today, we have many losses. Our world is larger than the *shtetl*, or Jewish village in Eastern Europe, where relationships were clearly defined. Our families are scattered far and wide, the media brings news of loss from parts of the globe we've never even heard of. And AIDS continues to ravage our world, our city, and our congregation. Perhaps when we stand all together, men and women supporting each other as we recite the *Kaddish,* we wonder "Just who am I saying this for?" We don't always have the narrow focus of one loss, we don't always have 11 months to grieve without another loss. And yet *Kaddish* gives us time to experience our memories, personal, communal, painful and joyous, too. The strange words can be a meditation as we reaffirm our faith in God, and reclaim this ritual as a tradition for our times.

A few weeks ago, I attended a memorial service for someone who died of AIDS. He was 23 years old when I met him and 26 when he died. He came to services here sometimes. In keeping with the way he had lived his life, his memorial service was held in a sex club. We saw photos of him bald and naked posing in a graveyard. We watched a video of him camping it up in drag. We told wonderful, funny stories about him. But in the background a tape played of him chanting his Torah portion at his bar mitzvah. And in the quiet candlelit upstairs room of that sex club, 35 of us rose together to recite the *Kaddish* for him.

Now you may be thinking, "What good does it do me to go to a memorial service and say *Kaddish*? The pain doesn't go away so easily and I don't come to synagogue to say *Kaddish* all that often. Grief goes on a long time."

Marcel Proust wrote:

". . . There is no more ridiculous custom than the one that makes
you express sympathy once and for all on a given day to a person
whose sorrow will endure as long as his [or her] life. Such grief,
felt in such a way, is always 'present,' it is never too late to talk
about it, never repetitious to mention it again."

Judaism recognizes this. Each year on the anniversary of a death, we commemorate the yahrzeit, coming to synagogue, giving *tzedakah* donations, reciting *Kaddish*. Our ancestors found an additional opportunity to mourn by creating *Yizkor*, the memorial service for all the dead, which we observe at Congregation Sha'ar Zahav twice a year. This is a time to reflect, to let the mind wander, to say a personal prayer for each person who comes to mind in our memory.

Now you may be thinking, "Won't these rituals encourage me to dwell on my grief?" On the contrary, by providing structure for our memories and our grief, Judaism helps us to find a way to remember without feeling so much pain. Our memories can become a legacy, reminding us how much we've learned about life from those who are no longer living, allowing them to "illuminate for us the path."

I've been working with people with AIDS for nine years now, and during that time I've lost several personal friends as well. Sometimes when someone I've become close to is dying, I ask myself the same question I asked with the first person I knew. When this person dies, will I be able to go on? Will I have the strength to open my heart again, so soon, to someone new? And what I've found has been new strength, strength renewed by Jewish tradition and practice, that says yes, I can go out and love some more.

Rabbi Chaim Stern wrote:

.   'Tis a fearful thing

to love what death can touch.

A fearful thing
to love, to hope, to dream, to be –

to be,
and oh, to lose.

A thing for fools, this,

and a holy thing,

a holy thing
to love.

LOOKING BACK

For your life has lived in me,
your laugh once lifted me.
your word was gift to me.

To remember this brings painful joy.

'Tis a human thing, love,
a holy thing, to love
what death can touch.

Acknowledgments

I wish to thank Abby Kovalsky for bringing me to the National AIDS Memorial Grove recently for a commemoration of 40 years since the beginning of the AIDS epidemic, which led me back to these writings and memories.

I am deeply grateful for the expert editorial eye and wisdom of Betsy Bannerman; the beautiful cover painted by Joe Bailey, a friend and former housemate from the early days; the photo by my sister, Erika Opper, as well as her willingness to get involved with this project; the kind words of Lisa Horowitz and Stuart Feinhor; and the helpful support and encouragement of Tony Tepper, Beth Krackov, Barbara Pastorello, Amy Barron, Jenny Andrus, Janet Parker, Susan Kahn, and Nitza Agam

I will never forget the love, comfort, and support both my parents offered during the challenging years I worked with people with AIDS.

Author Biography

In 1983 Jody Opper Reiss began volunteering as an AIDS case manager for the Whitman-Walker Clinic in Washington, DC and later served as the clinic's first social work intern as she was studying for her Master of Social Work degree at the University of Maryland in Baltimore. Upon graduation in 1985, she was among the first professionals trained to be HIV-antibody test counselors, and worked in the Health Departments in Montgomery and Prince Georges Counties in Maryland as well as at the Gay and Lesbian Center in Baltimore. In 1986, she joined the Department of Social Services in Prince Georges County, providing in-service trainings on AIDS for the department and eventually becoming lead social worker of an AIDS unit run in coordination with the Health Department. During this time, she also worked as a consultant for the National Institute of Drug Abuse, providing AIDS workshops for the staff of methadone clinics.

At the end of 1989, Jody returned to her native San Francisco, and for the next 10 years served as AIDS Project Coordinator for Jewish Family and Children's Services in San Francisco, a multi-faceted program providing counseling, case management, and support for Jewish clients with AIDS and their loved ones, along with two volunteer programs and the "Putting a Face to AIDS" speakers' bureau and education program.

In 1997 she developed and taught a six-month course for HIV case managers from 30 agencies for the San Francisco Department of Public Health, and from 1995 to 1997 she taught the course "Social Work with People with AIDS" at the School of Social Work at San Francisco State University. In 2000, Jody served as a medical social worker for, among other patients, those with AIDS at Davies Medical Center in San Francisco.

Following 18 years of work in the AIDS field, Jody entered private psychotherapy practice. She worked with individuals and groups, specializing in bipolar disorder and addictions. She retired from private practice in 2016. Still living in San Francisco, she now engages in various volunteer and political activities and sings with the Threshold Choir, which sings to ill and dying patients in a variety of settings.

www.ingramcontent.com/pod-product-compliance
Lightning Source LLC
Chambersburg PA
CBHW030406290526
45785CB00004B/1916